WHAT IS CEREBRAL PALSY?

A simple explanation of a complex diagnosis

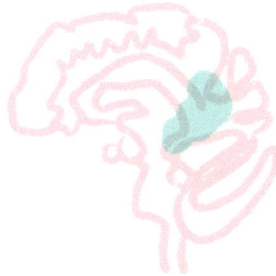

Written by Hailey Adkisson
Illustrated by Kelsey Diaz

First printing, 2025.

SIMPLY COMPLEX stories

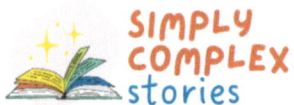

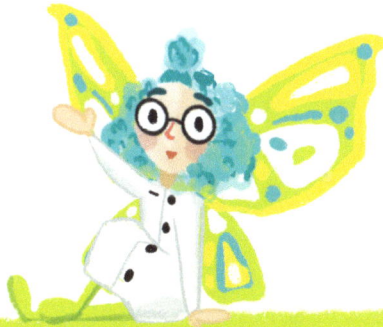

To those with Cerebral Palsy (CP) –
be unapologetically you. You are
seen and you are valued.

And to those parents and caregivers
with a newly diagnosed child– you
are not alone.

A huge thank you to the dozens of people who reviewed this book and provided feedback including parents/caregivers to children with CP, doctors and therapists that work alongside people with CP, and most importantly, the many adults and children with CP who provided extremely valuable insight. Without you, this book would not be possible.

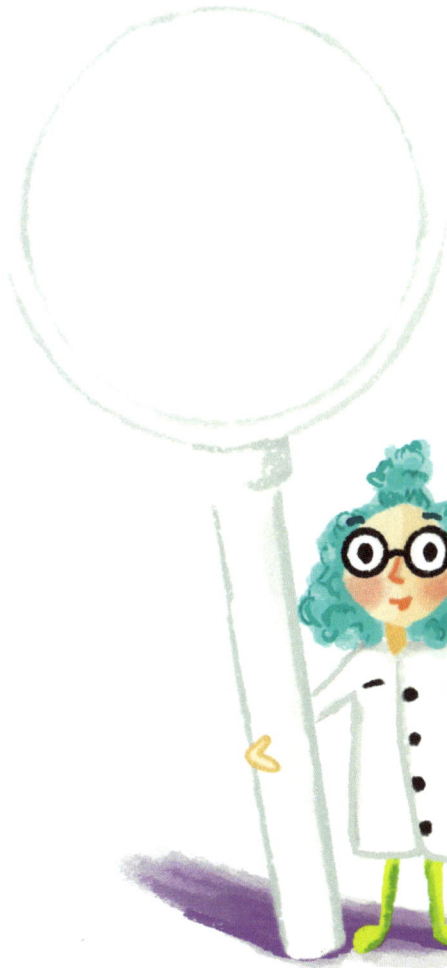

Hi! My name is Effie, and today I'm going to talk to you about cerebral palsy.

Did you know that you have over 600 muscles in your body? Muscles help you sit up tall, run fast, wave at friends, chew your food, and even help you breathe.

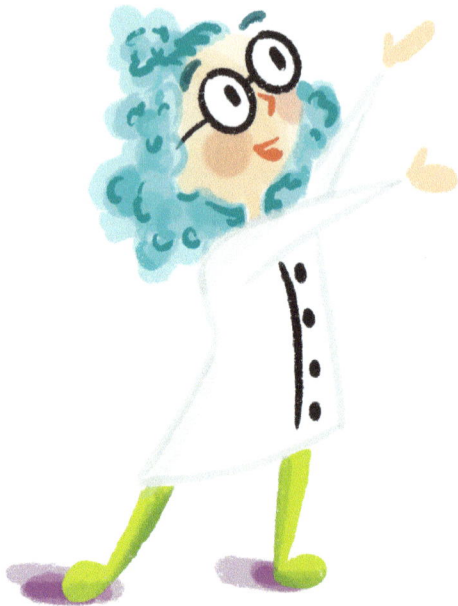

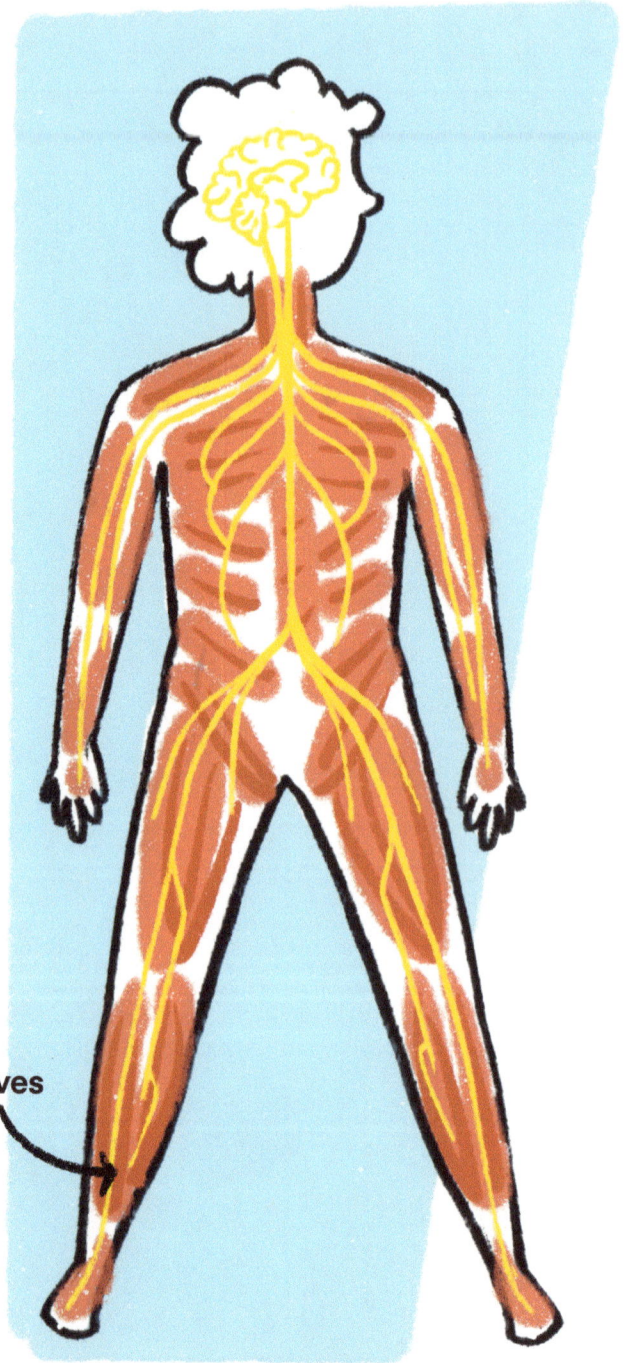

Nerves

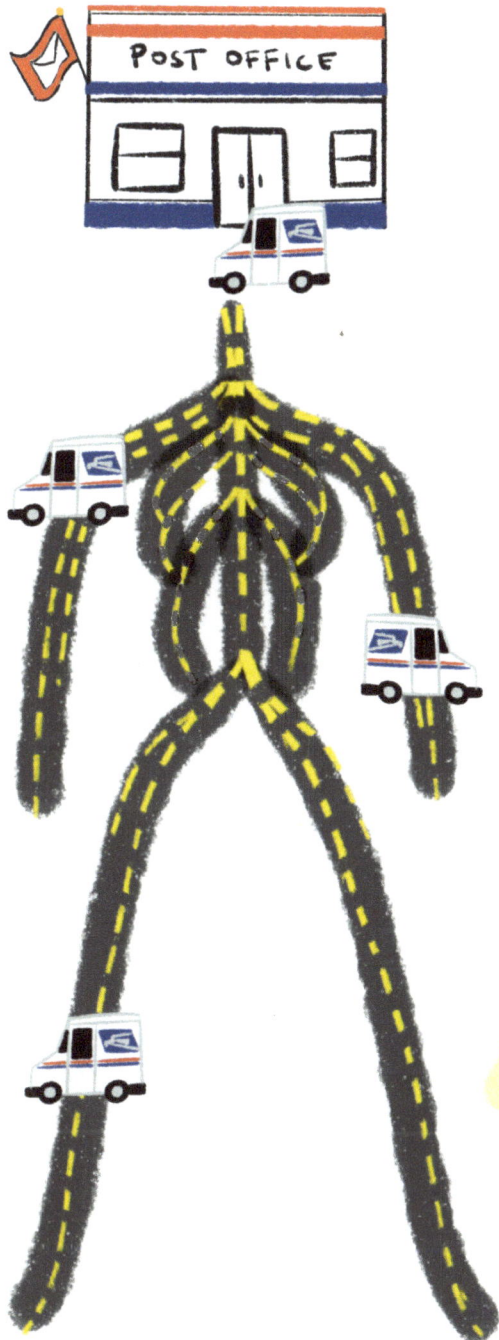

Your brain tells your muscles when and how to move. To do this, your brain sends messages throughout your entire body along "roads" called nerves.

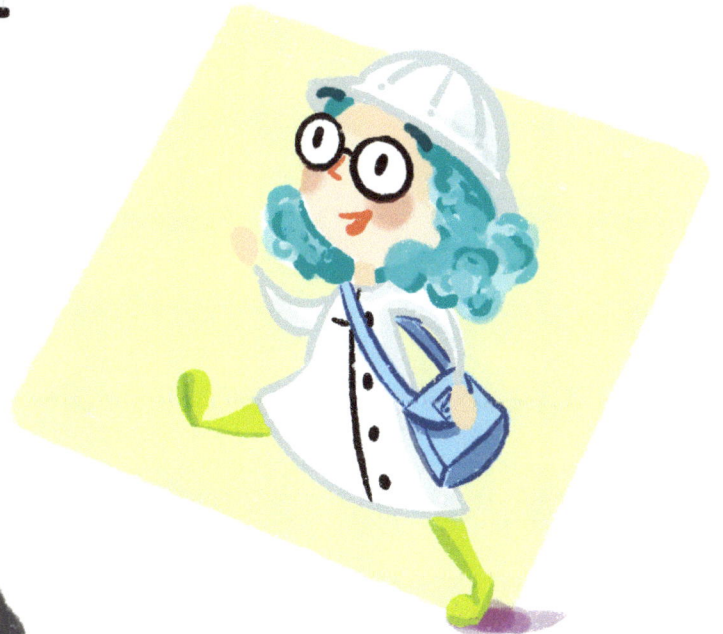

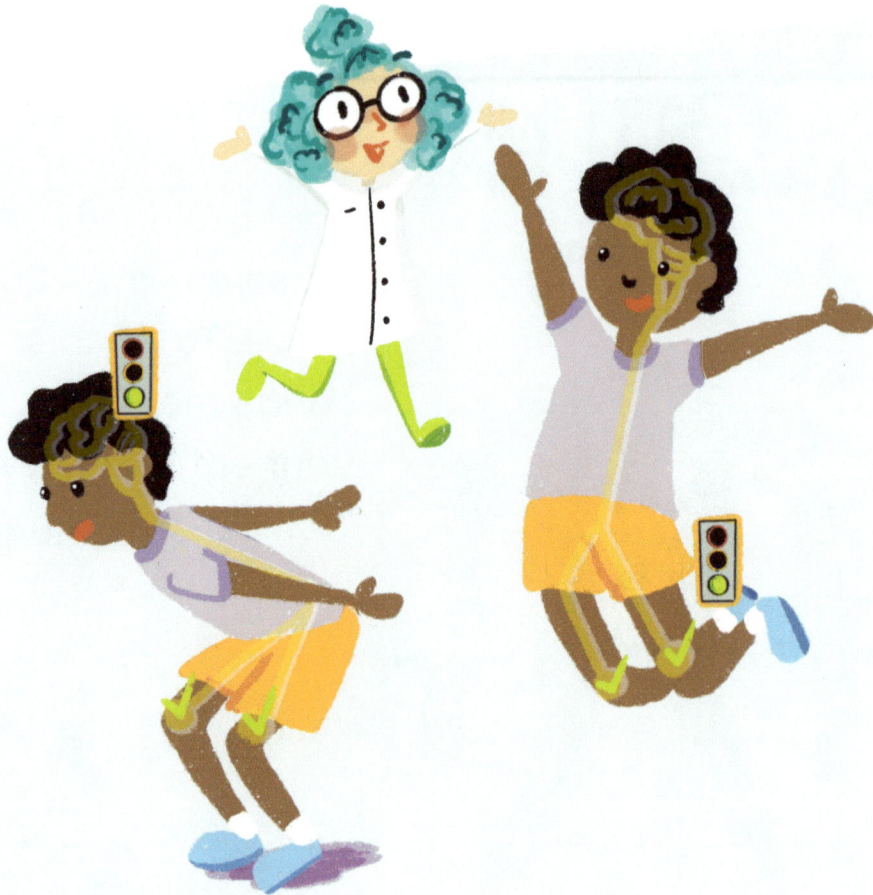

Different parts of your brain control different muscles. For example, if you want to jump, your brain will send a message through your nerves to your leg muscles to help you jump!

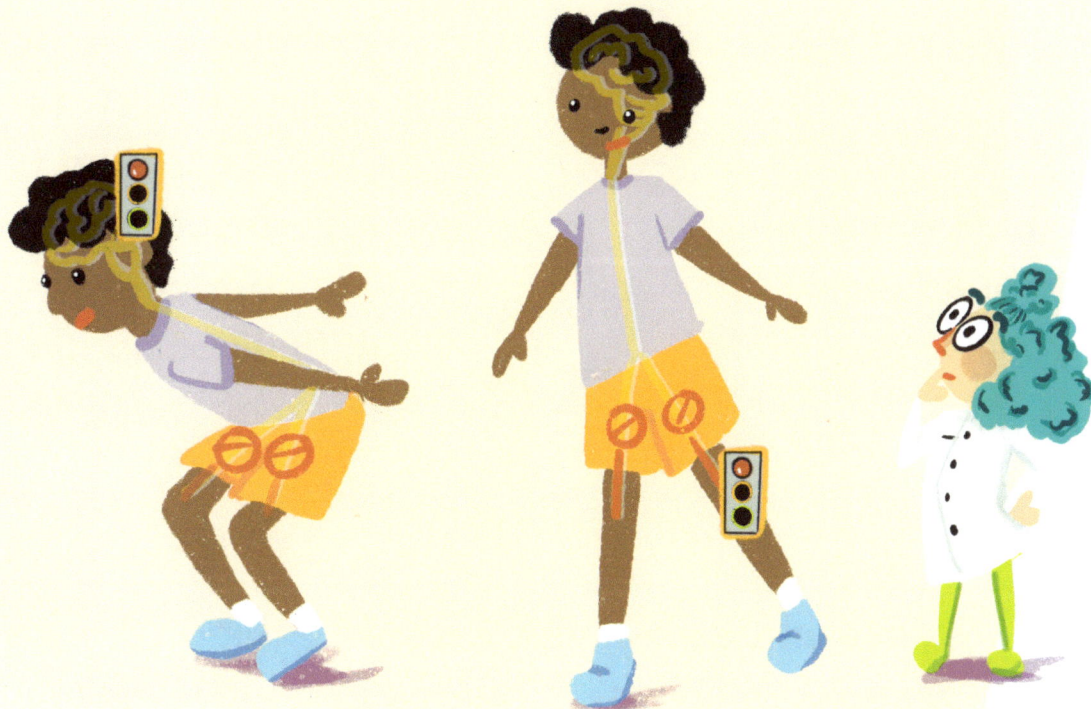

But sometimes, the message from a person's brain can get disrupted, making it difficult for that person to control their muscles. This disruption is called cerebral palsy (or CP for short).

"Cerebral" (SER-ee-bruhl) means something involving your brain.

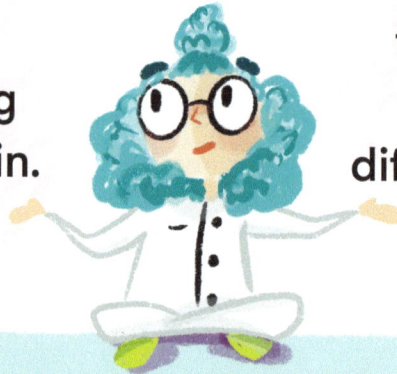

"Palsy" (PAWL-zee) is a medical word used to describe when someone has difficulties controlling their muscles.

So, cerebral palsy is a medical condition that makes it difficult for someone to control their muscles because of a change in their brain.

Typical: speedy message delivery

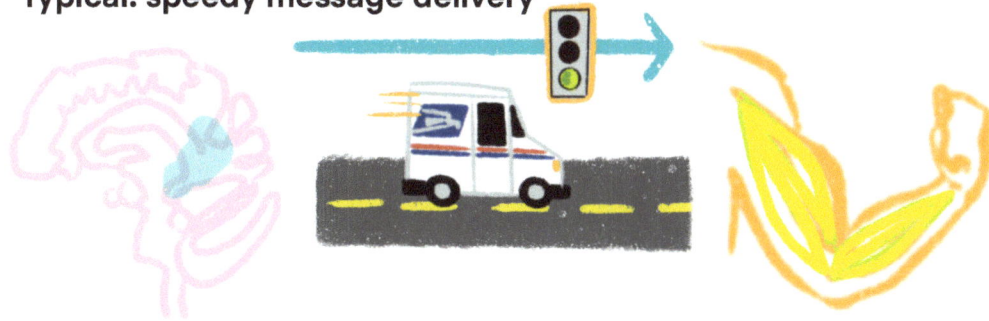

CP: messaged delivery disrupted

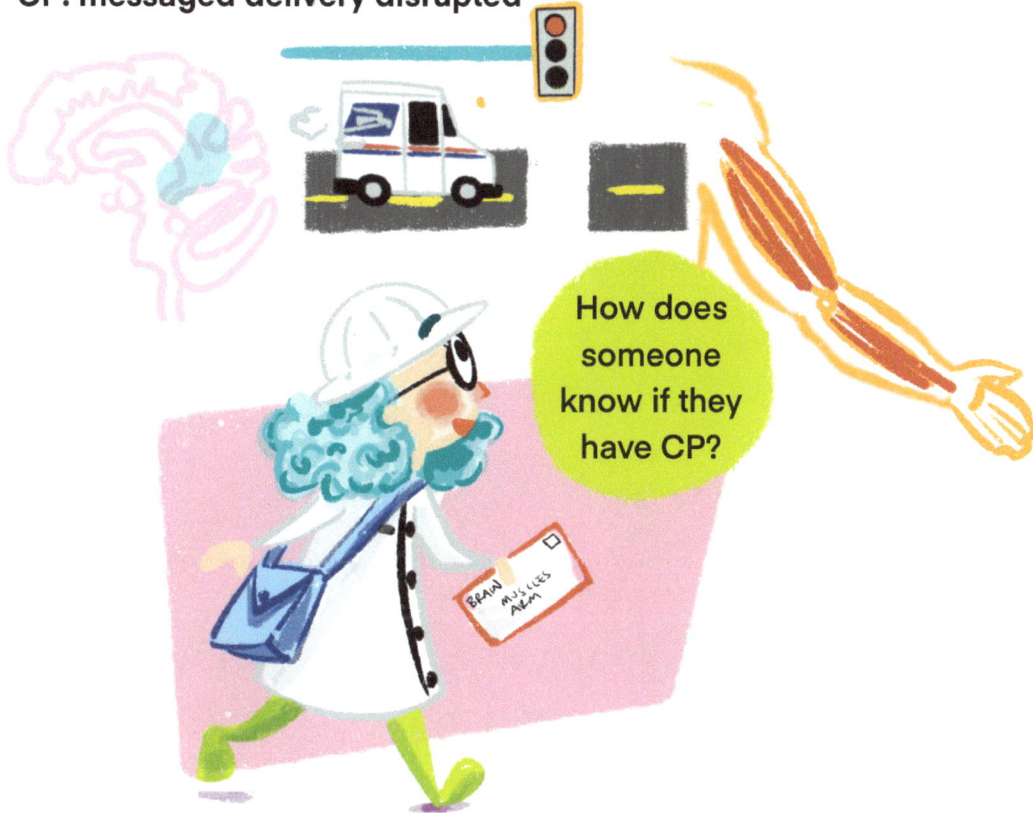

How does someone know if they have CP?

Most people learn they have CP before they turn two. First, they visit a doctor that studies the brain and nerves. This doctor is called a neurologist (nur-AH-luh-jist).

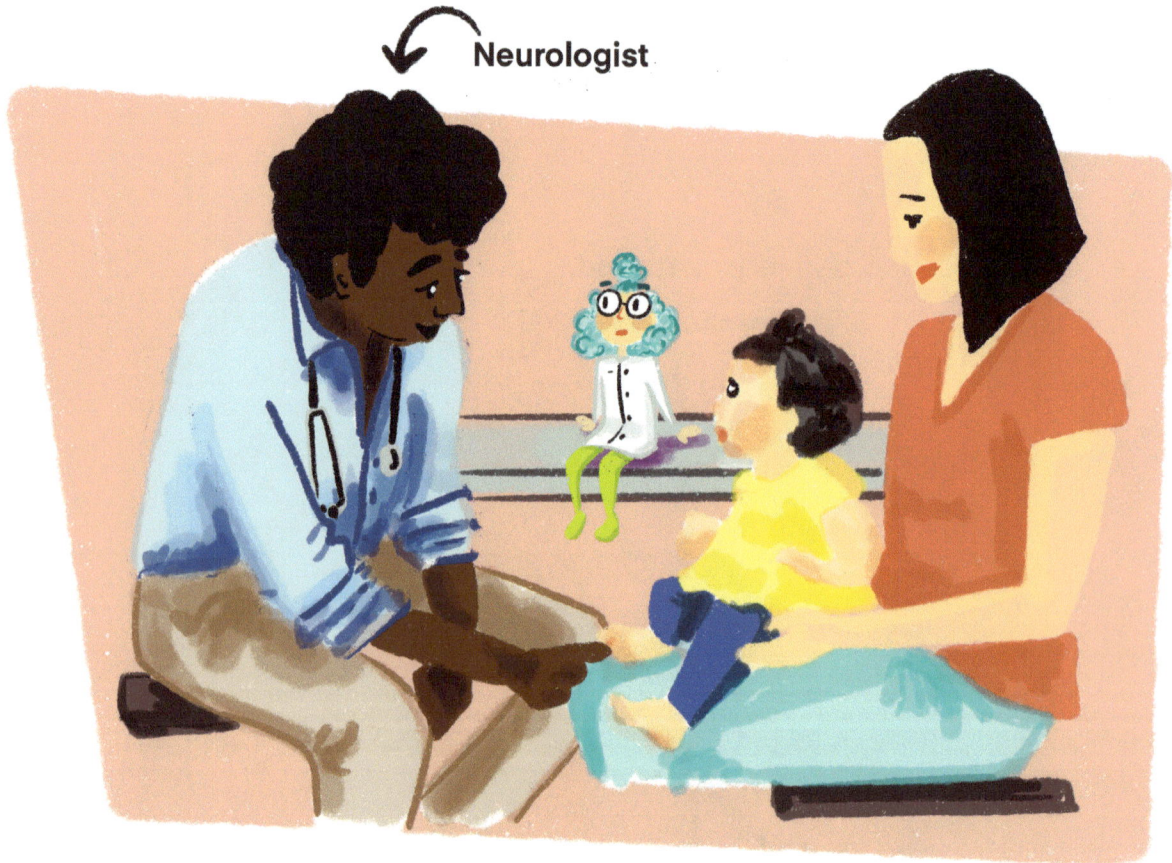

Neurologist

The neurologist will look at how the person moves and ask about any concerns their parents or caregivers might have.

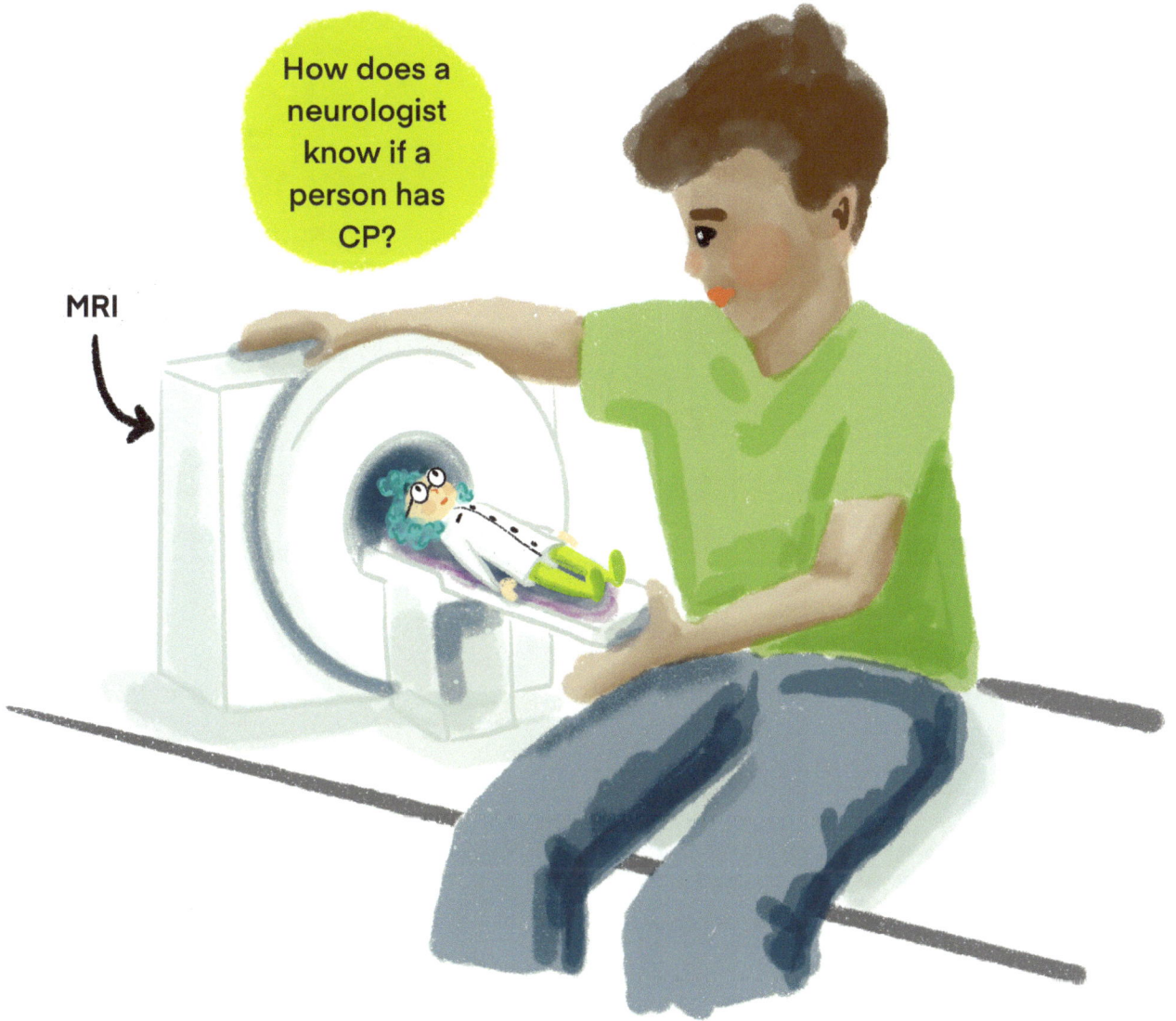

The neurologist may want to take pictures of their brain using a big machine called an MRI.

How does a neurologist know if a person has CP?

MRI

Just like everyone looks and acts differently, CP can look and act differently too.

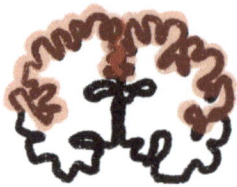

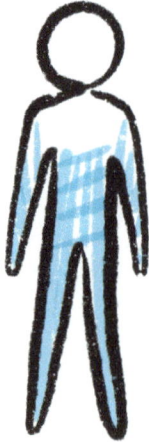

When CP affects both arms and both legs it's called:

Quadriplegia (kwah-druh-PLEE-gee-uh)

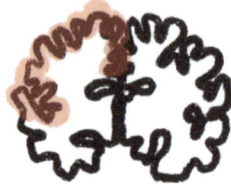

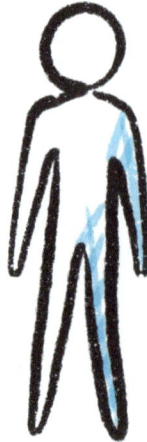

When CP affects one arm/one leg on the same side it's called:

Hemiplegia (hem-uh-PLEE-gee-uh)

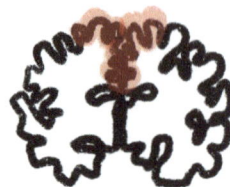

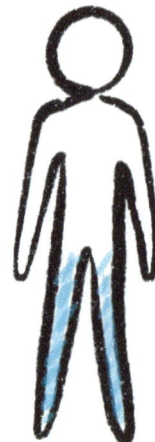

When CP affects only legs it's called:

Diplegia (dye-PLEE-gee-uh)

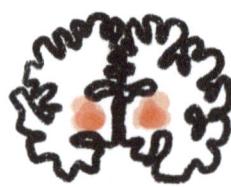

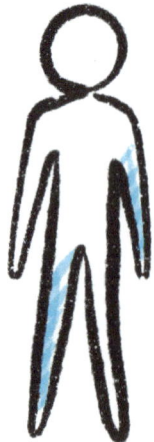

When CP affects only one leg or only one arm it's called:

Monoplegia (mon-uh-PLEE-gee-uh)

Spastic (SPAS-tik)

Some forms of CP cause muscles to be stiff and tight

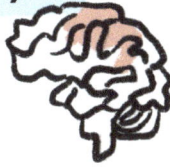

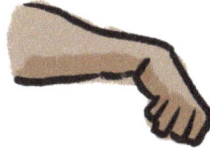

Dyskinetic (dis-kih-NET-ik)

Other forms of CP cause someone to move/twist their arms or legs even if they don't want to, or cause muscles to get "stuck" in painful positions.

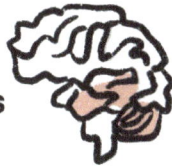

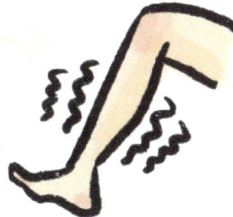

Ataxic (uh-TAK-sik)

Some forms of CP cause people to have difficulties with balance or moving parts of their body smoothly

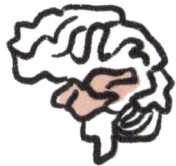

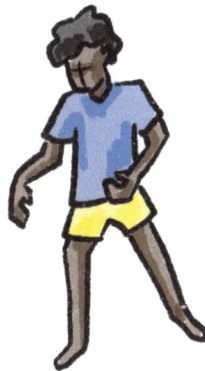

Hypotonic (hy-puh-TON-ik)

Other forms of CP cause muscles to get too relaxed and loose

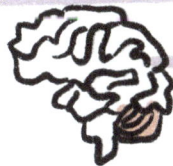

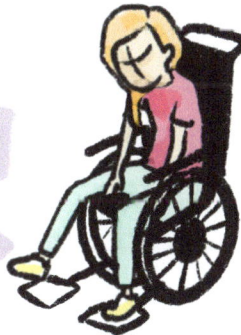

Once the neurologist finds out what parts of the body are impacted, they look at how the muscles in those body parts move.
Some forms of CP have a combination of more than one type, when this happens it's called Mixed CP.

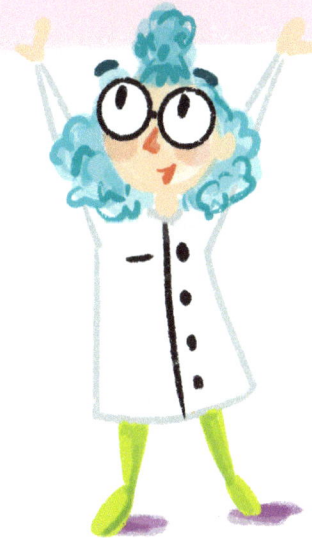

11

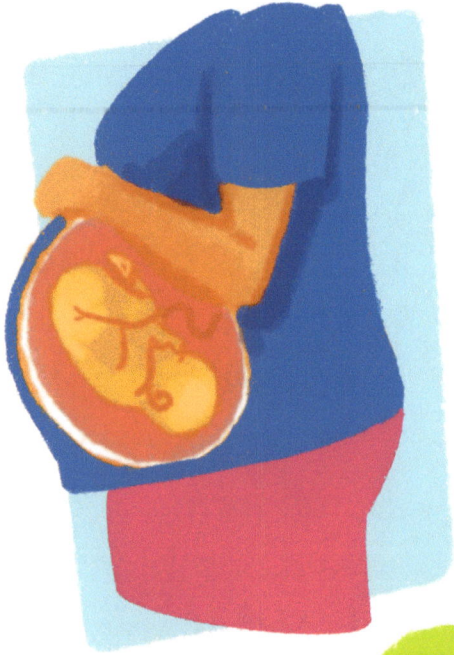

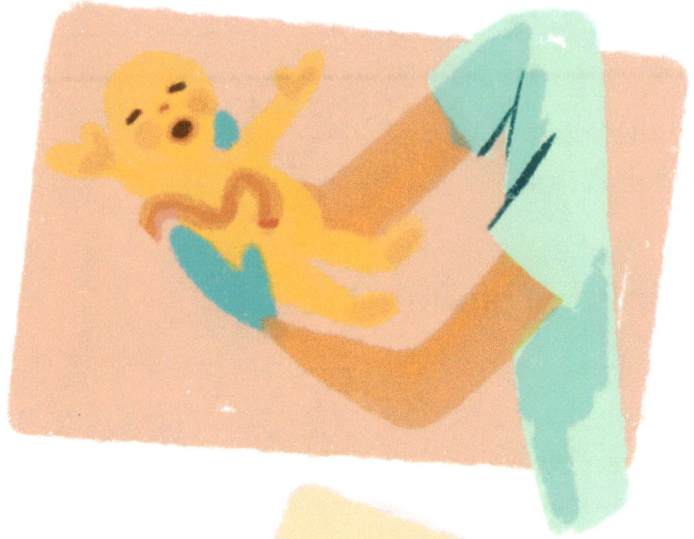

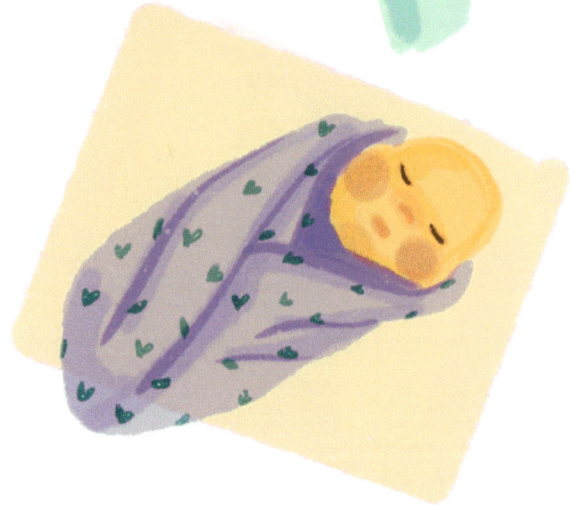

What
causes
CP?

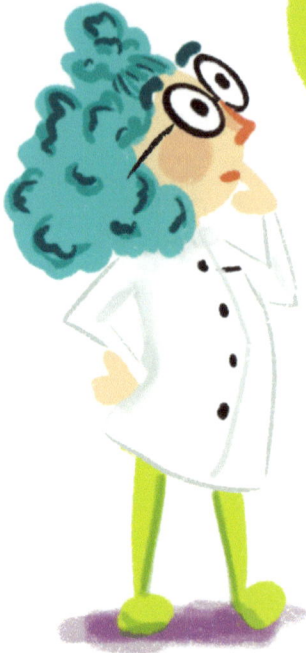

CP is caused by a change in how the brain grows or due to an injury to the brain that happened before birth, during, or shortly after a baby is born.

When a baby is growing inside a uterus, their brain is growing too. For some people, their brains grew in a way that is different from a typical brain. Many of these differences can cause CP.

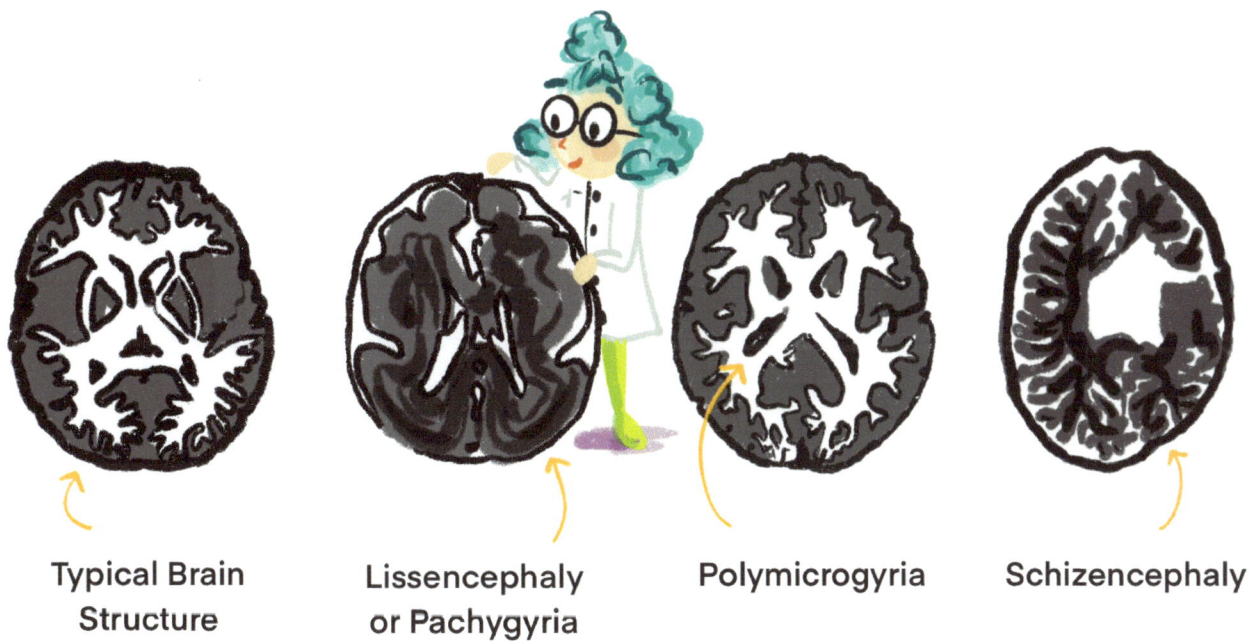

Typical Brain Structure

Lissencephaly or Pachygyria

Polymicrogyria

Schizencephaly

Another cause of CP is if a baby's brain doesn't have enough oxygen. Our body needs oxygen to stay alive. Oxygen is what helps us breathe and also helps to keep our brains running smoothly.

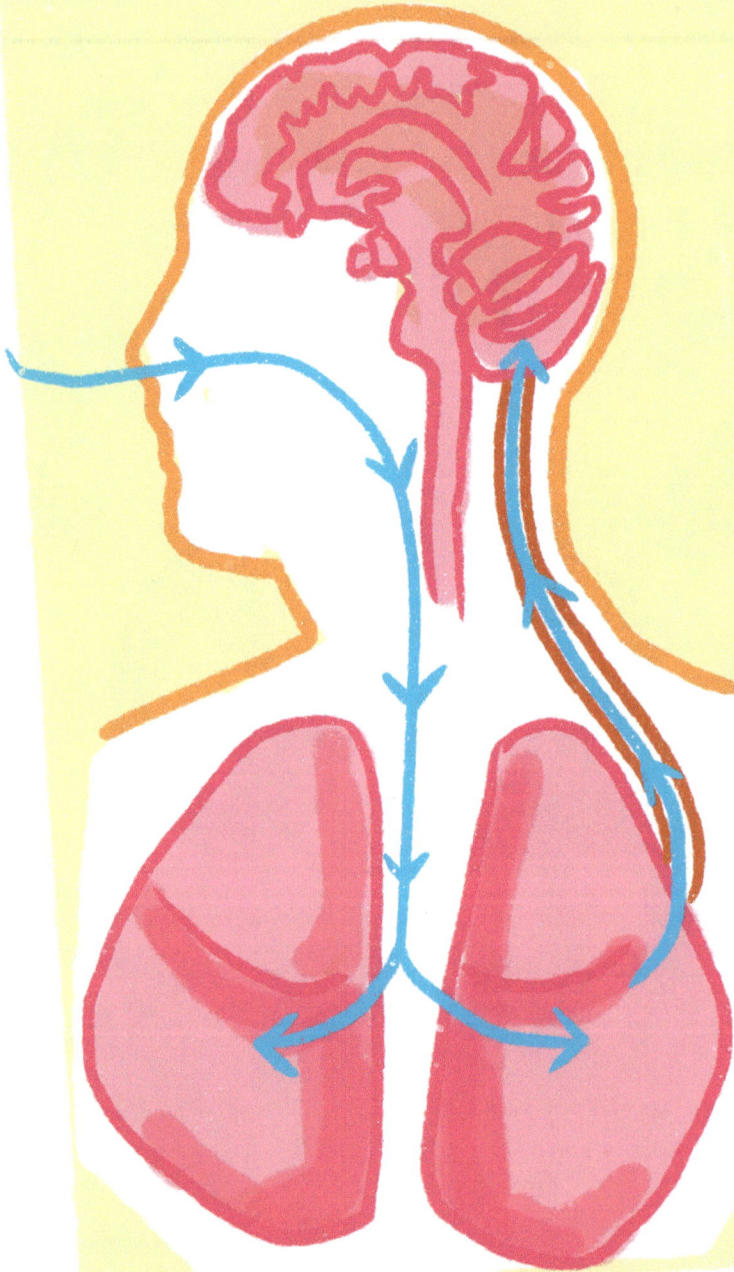

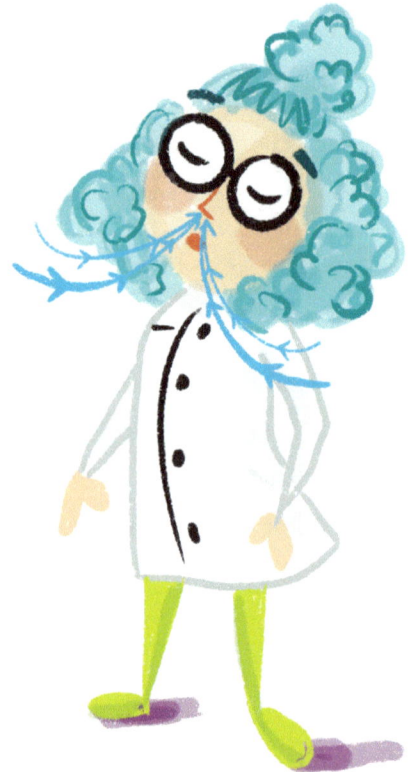

How does oxygen get to our brain? Through blood! Blood sends oxygen to our brain, and throughout our entire body, by traveling through "pipes" called blood vessels.

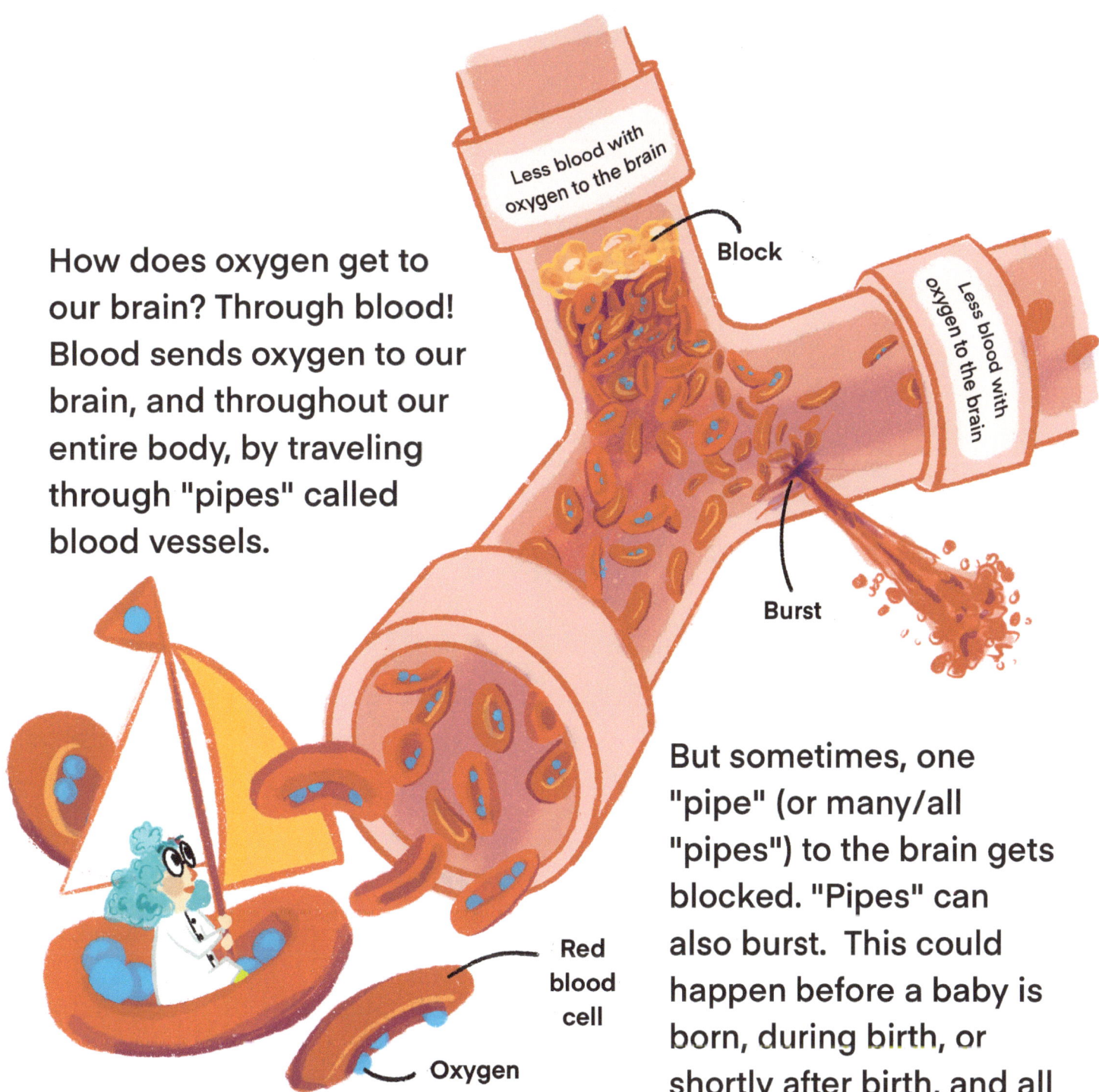

Less blood with oxygen to the brain

Block

Less blood with oxygen to the brain

Burst

Red blood cell

Oxygen

But sometimes, one "pipe" (or many/all "pipes") to the brain gets blocked. "Pipes" can also burst. This could happen before a baby is born, during birth, or shortly after birth, and all can cause CP.

15

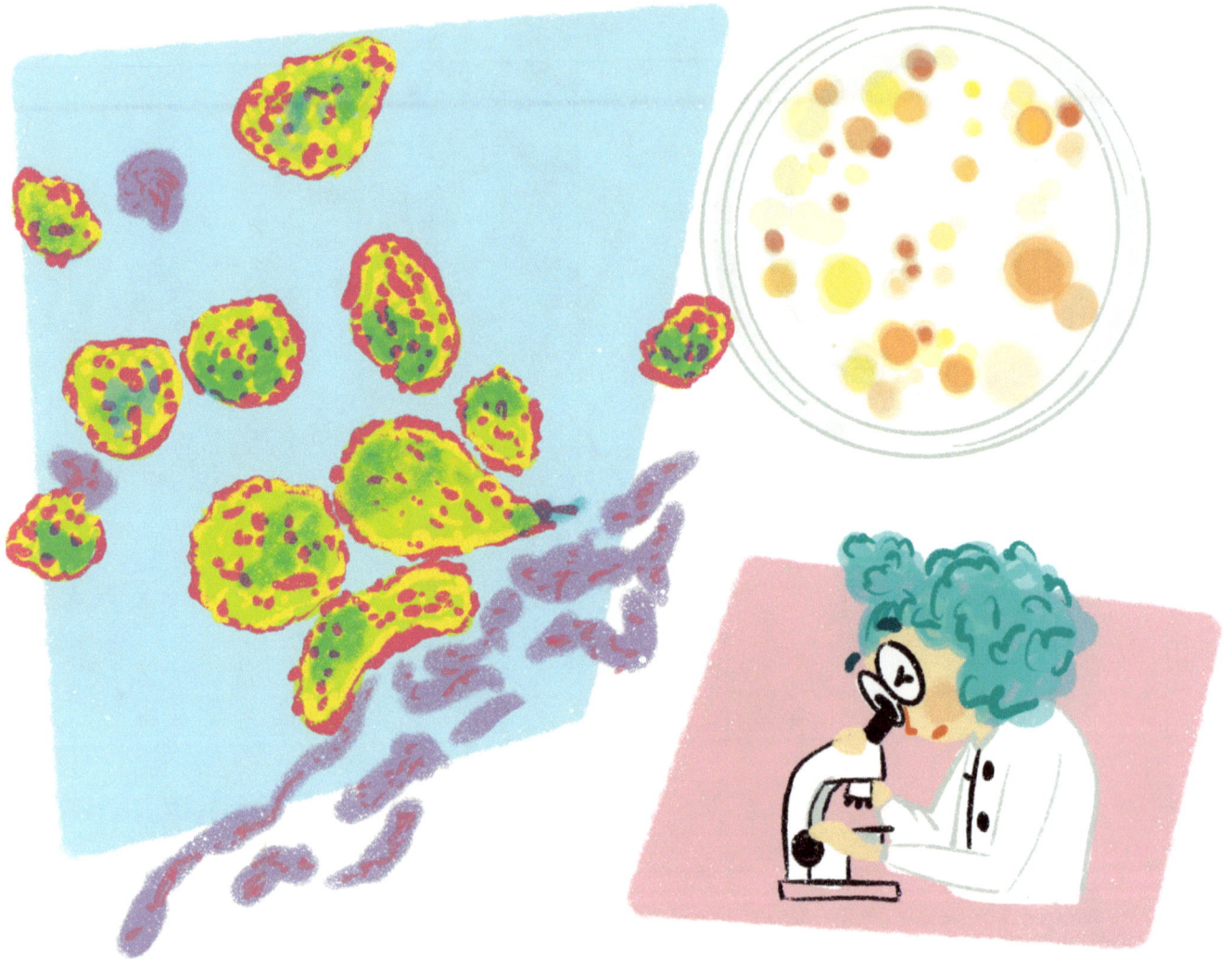

For some people, CP was caused because of germs. A baby can catch these germs before or after they are born. While not many germs cause CP, the ones that do are very dangerous because they can injure a baby's brain.

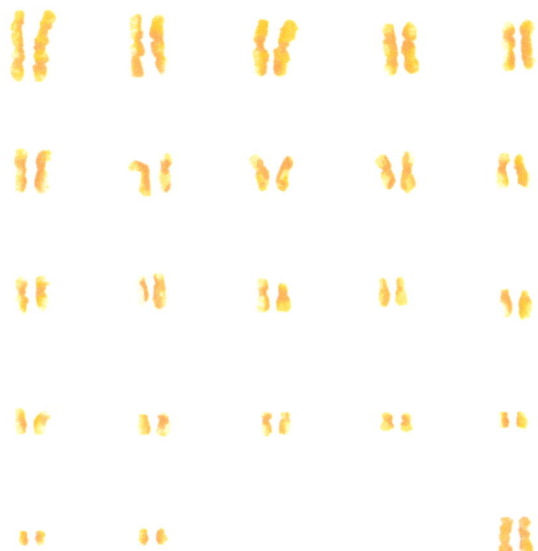

Another reason someone can have CP is a change in their genes. While J-E-A-N-S are pants you wear, G-E-N-E-S are like a set of instructions that helped make you YOU.

Chromosome

Cell

Gene

Genes decide what eye color you have, what hair color you have, and even how tall you will be. In some people, their instructions may have a rare change that cause CP.

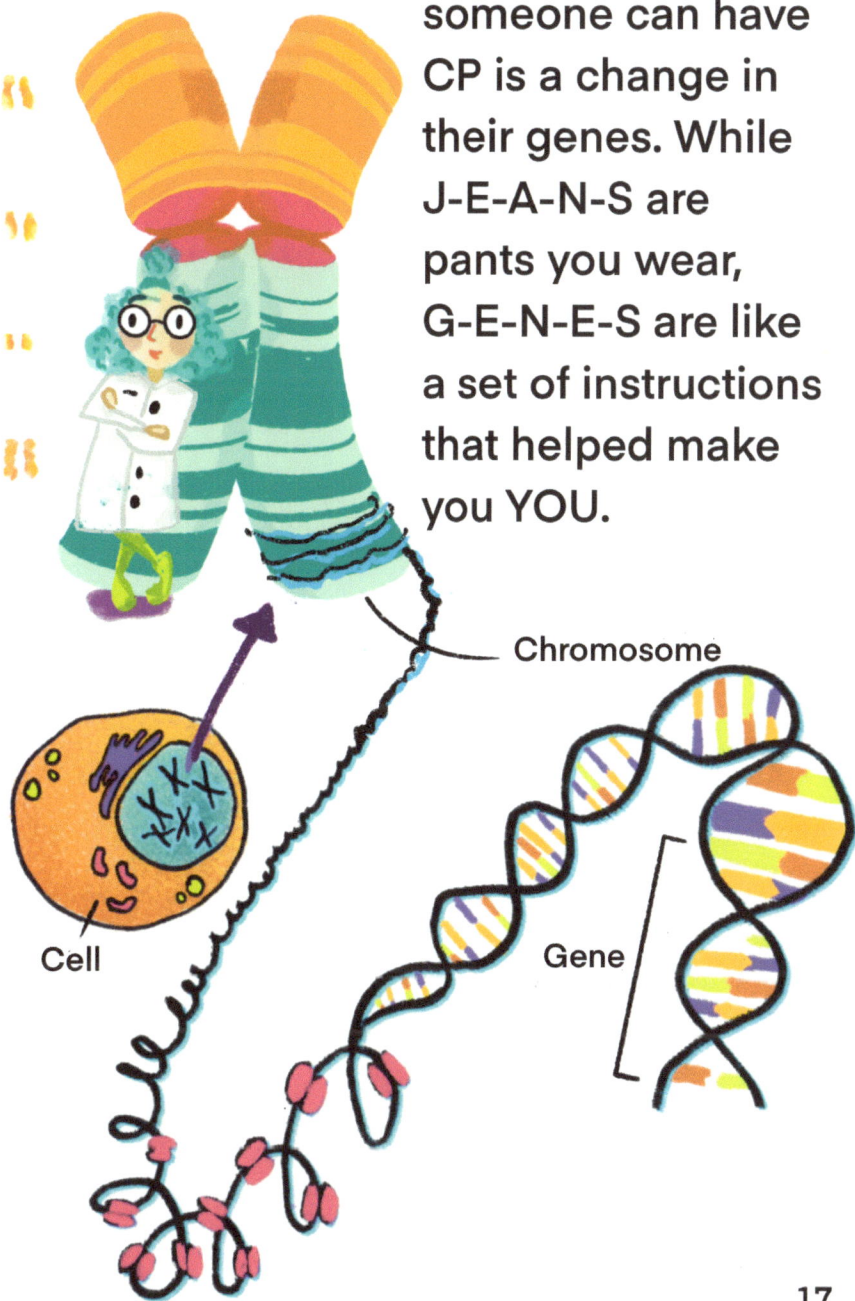

When a baby is born very early (called premature), their body and brain are very small and fragile. This makes a premature baby more likely to have CP.

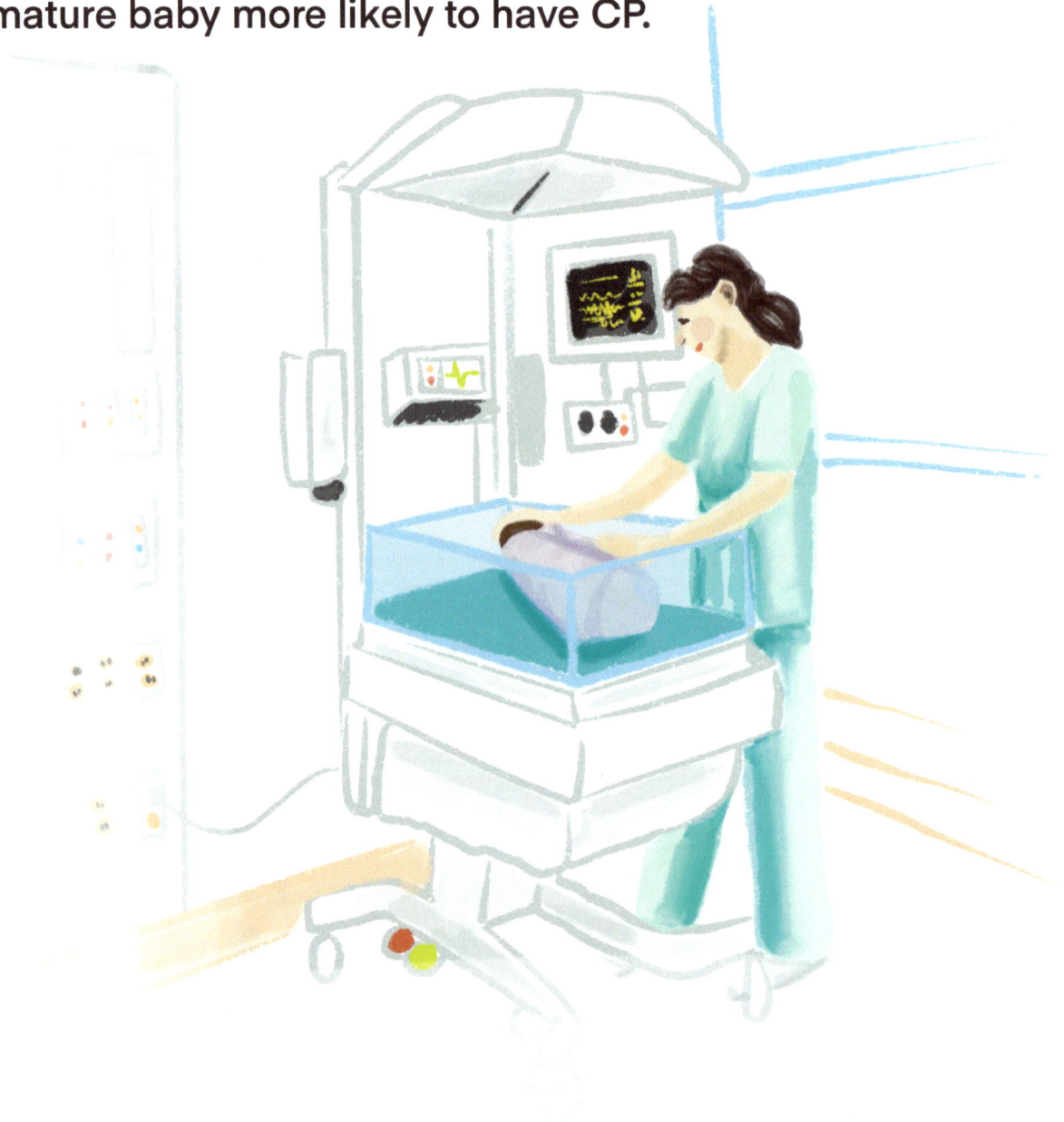

Sometimes, not even doctors can figure out the cause of a person's CP. That is why we need more people learning about CP and finding new causes.

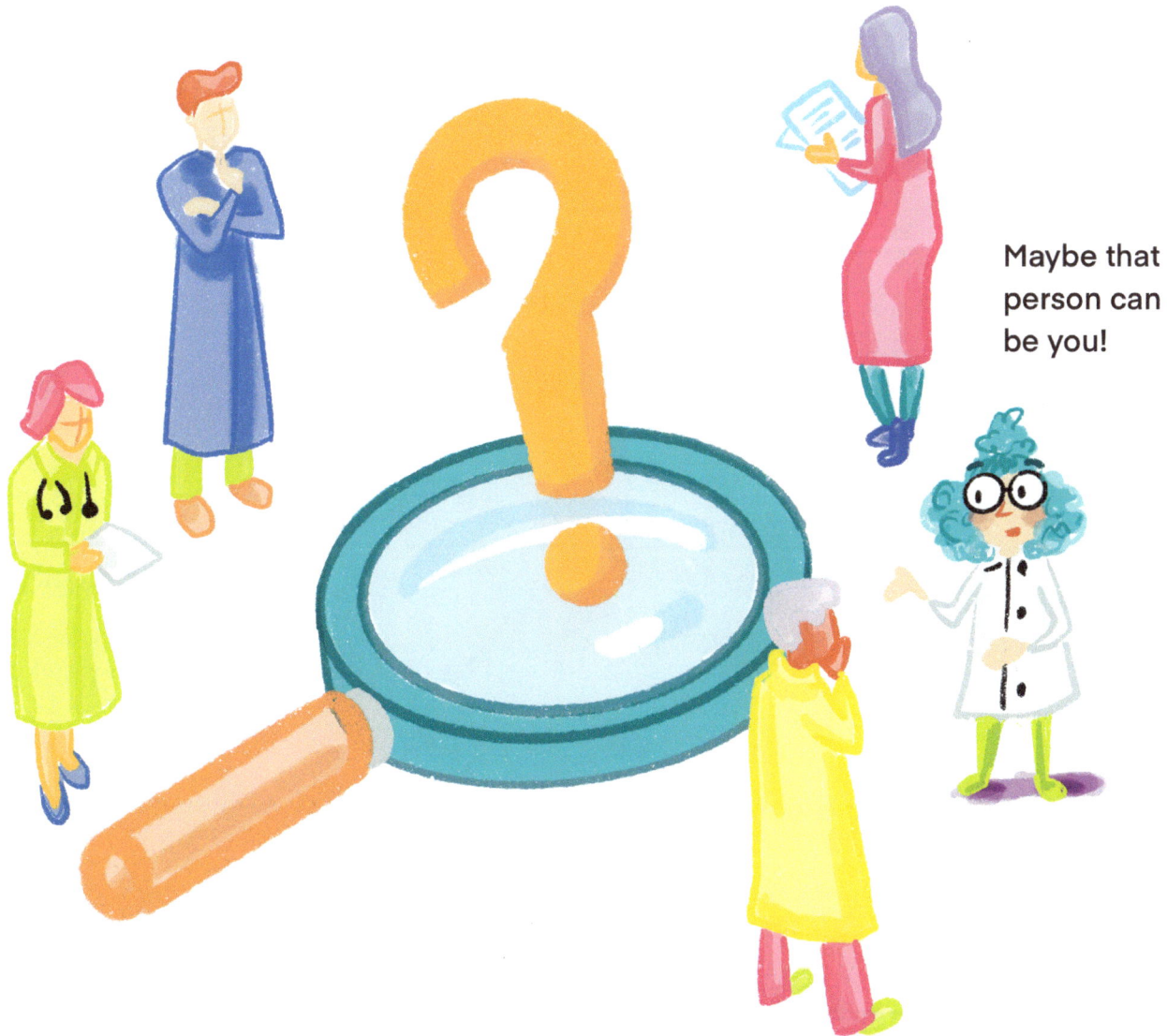

Maybe that person can be you!

There is no cure for CP, and that's okay! Many people with CP live very happy lives. They don't need to be fixed and you shouldn't feel sorry for them. However, there are things a person with CP can do to make life more comfortable.

Physical therapy can help people with CP learn exercises that help strengthen their muscles and move more easily.

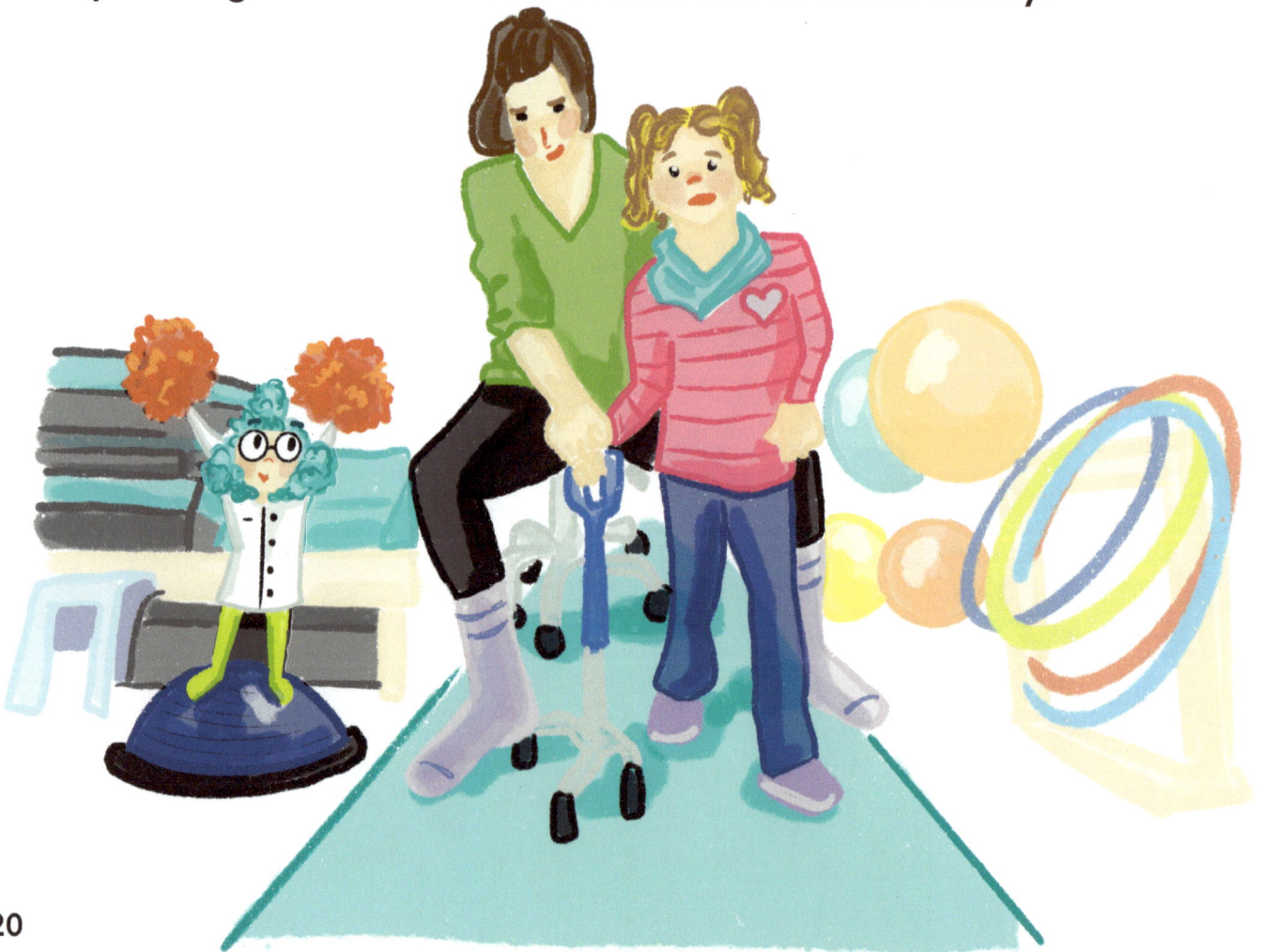

Occupational therapy can help people with CP learn to do everyday activities more easily like eating, getting dressed, writing, or playing with toys.

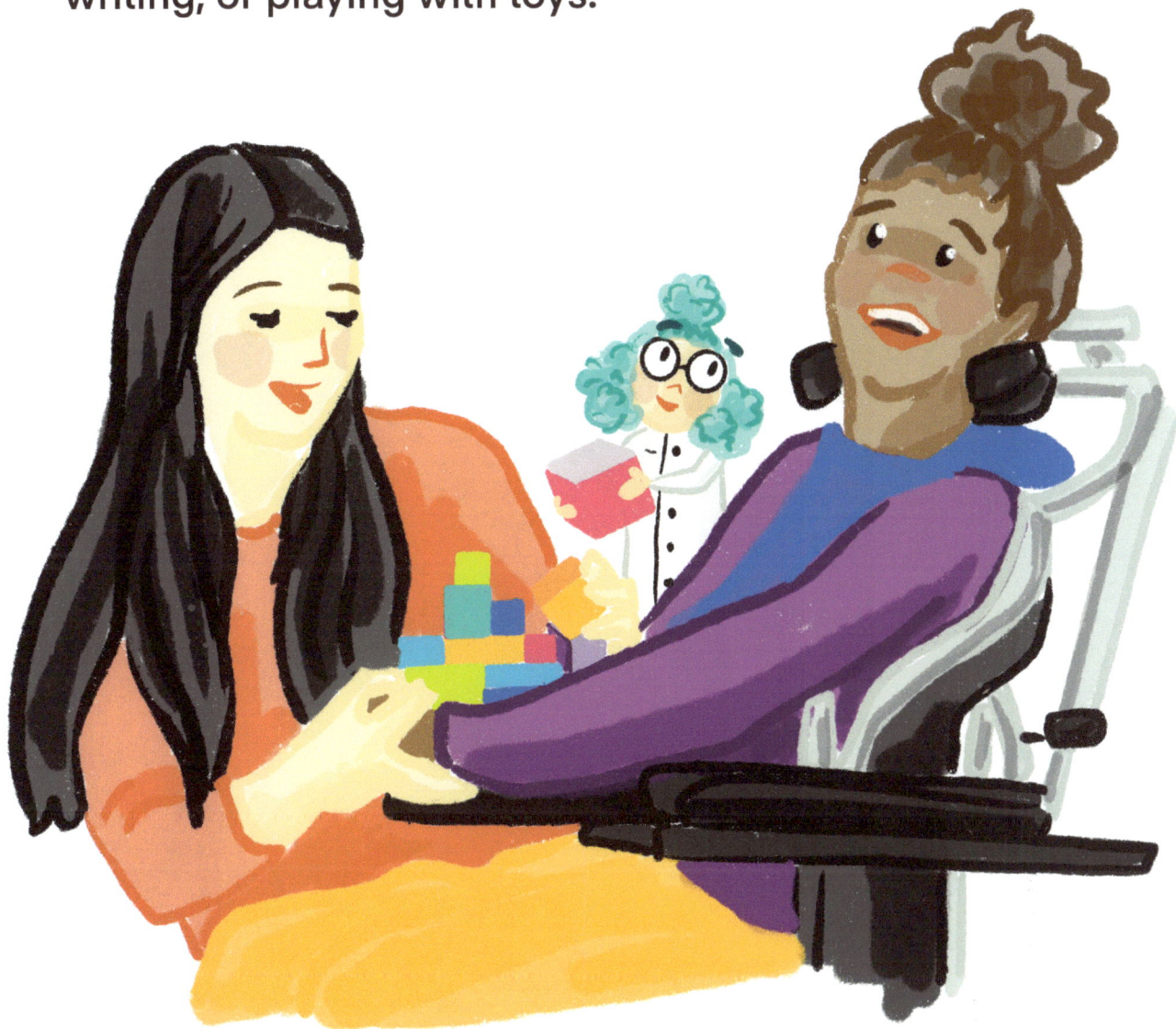

For some people with CP, their muscles can get very tight and difficult to move.

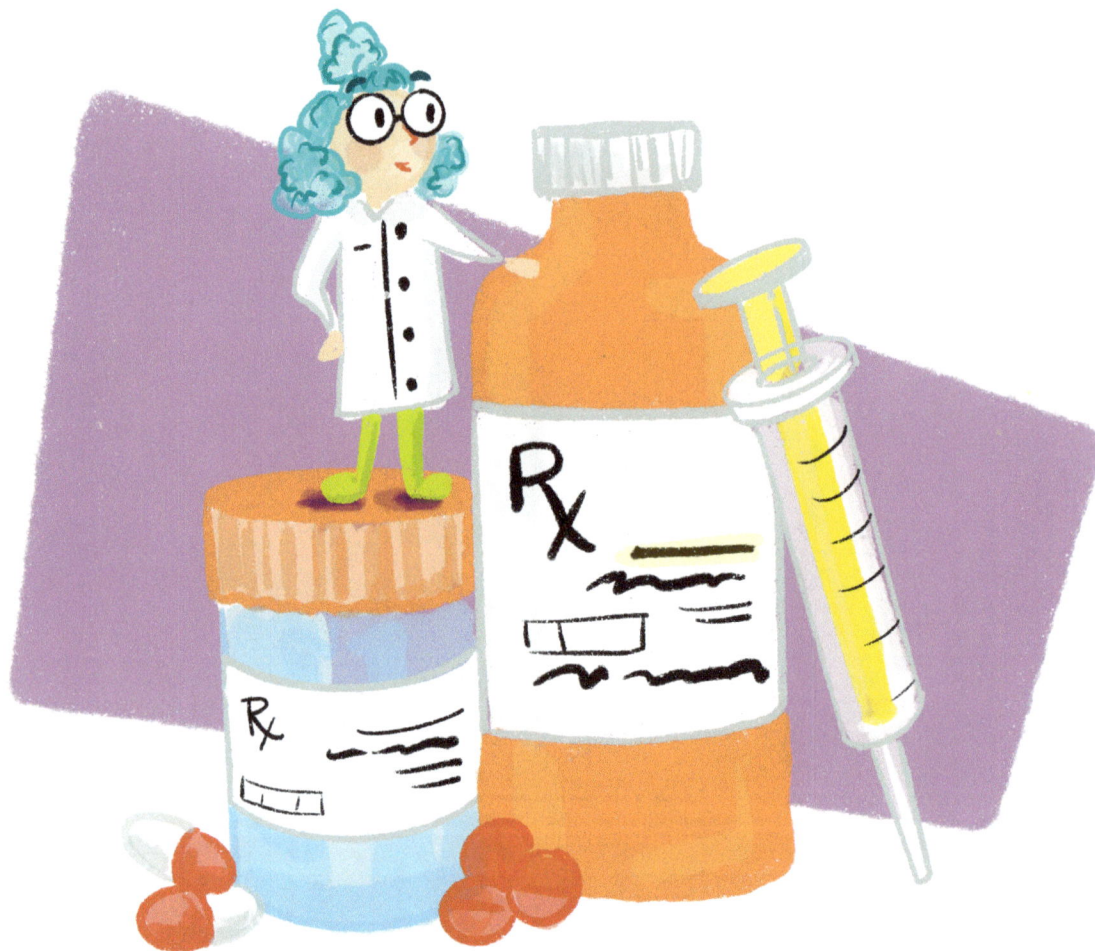

This can be painful and uncomfortable. Someone with CP may take medicine to help relax their muscles and make it easier to move and play.

People with CP may look or act differently from people without CP.

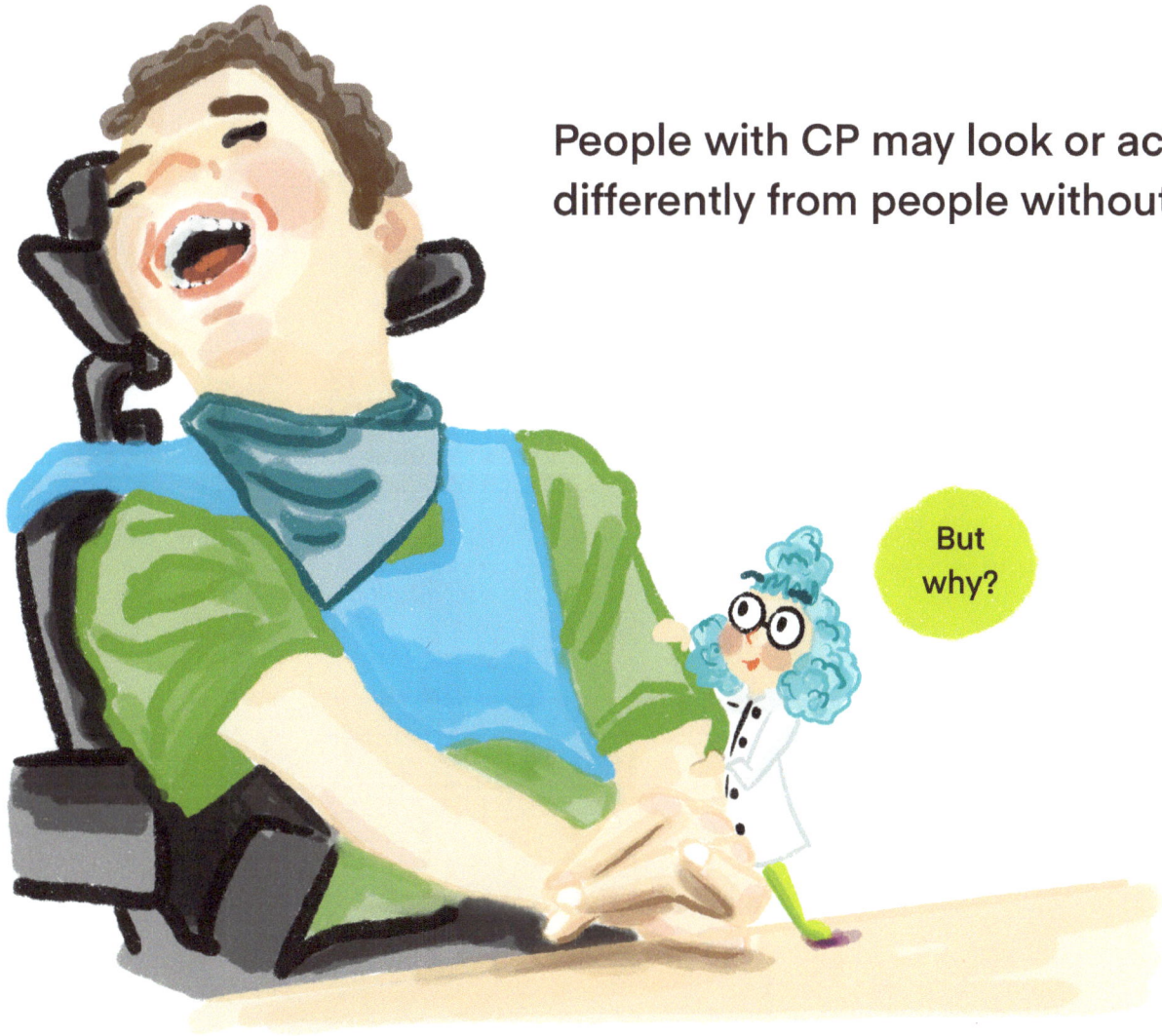

But why?

When a person has CP, parts of their brain are injured or changed, making it difficult to send messages to certain muscles. Where the injury is located in the brain determines what muscles are impacted.

If you see someone with CP using a wheelchair, walker, or cane, it may be because the part of their brain that helps them walk is injured.

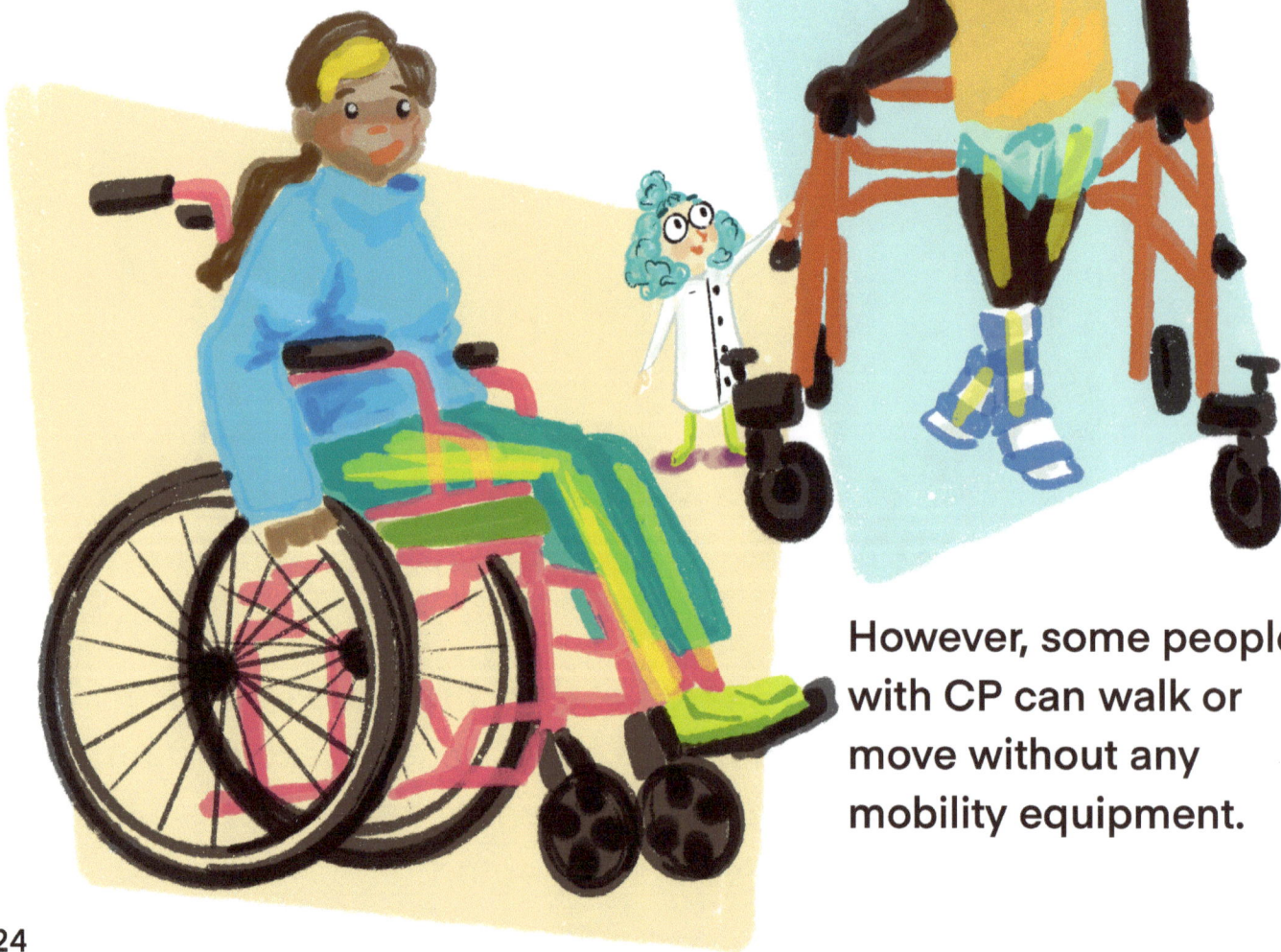

However, some people with CP can walk or move without any mobility equipment.

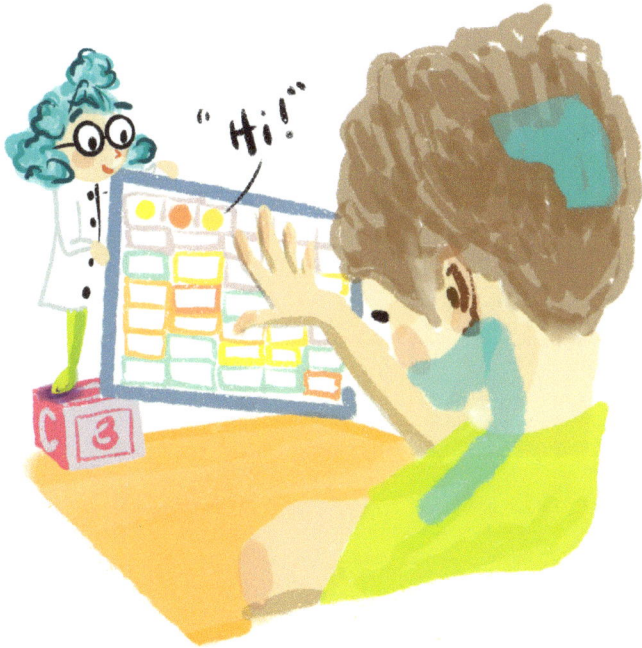

If you see someone with CP using a computer, buttons, or pictures to talk (called AAC), it may be because the part of their brain that controls speaking is injured.

If you see someone with CP eating through a feeding tube in their stomach instead of by mouth, it may be because the part of their brain that controls chewing and swallowing safely might be injured.

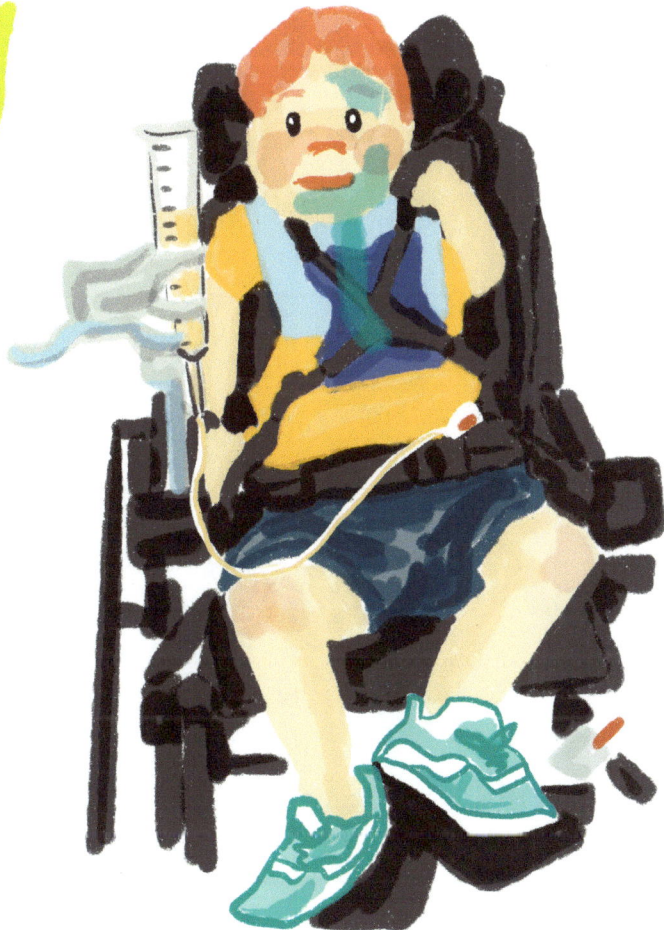

Some people with CP don't have noticeable differences. You may not know they have CP unless they choose to tell you. But no matter how someone walks, talks, moves, or eats, you should always treat people with kindness, never assume someone can't understand what you're saying, and always include them in activities.

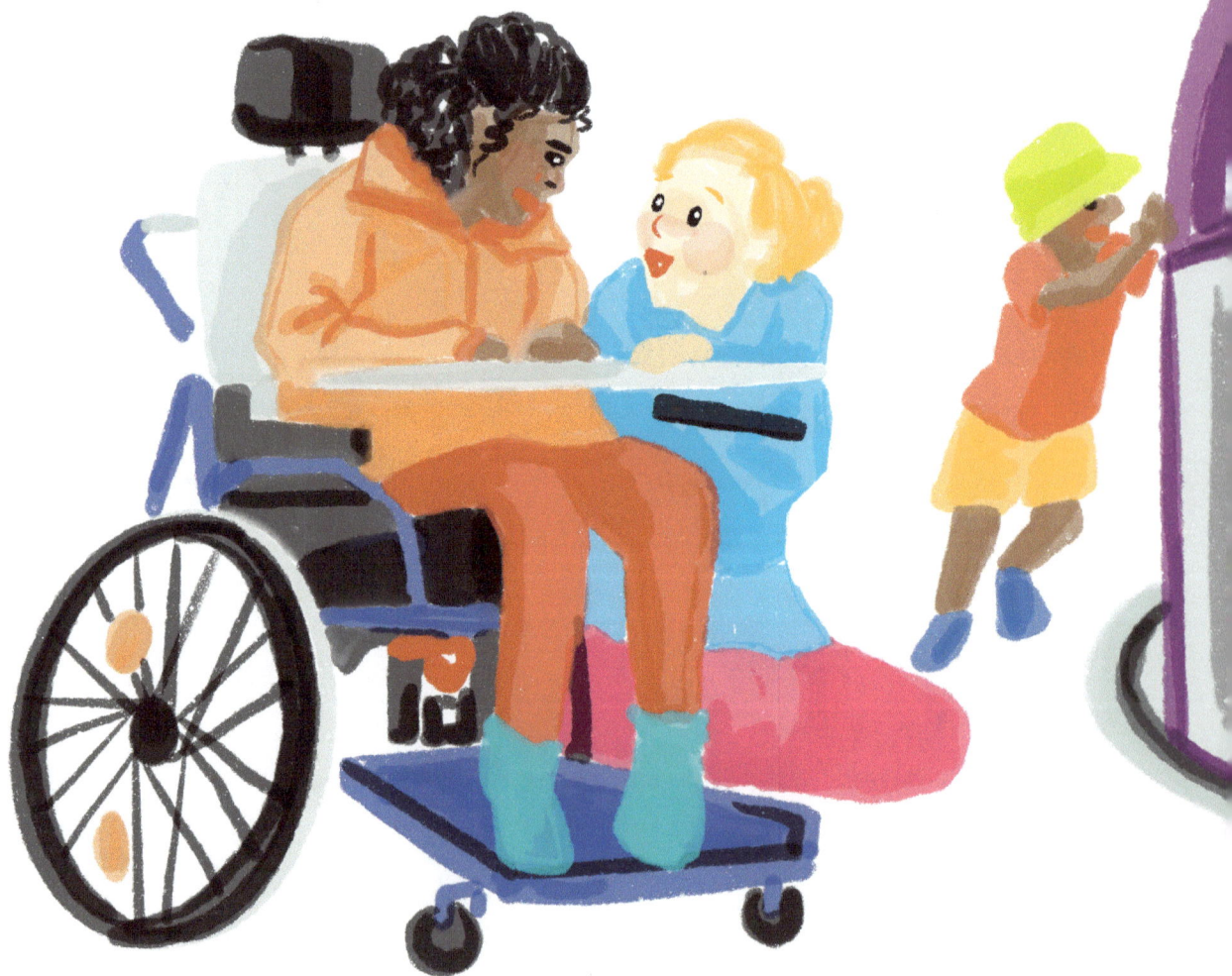

People with CP want to play and make friends just like everyone else!

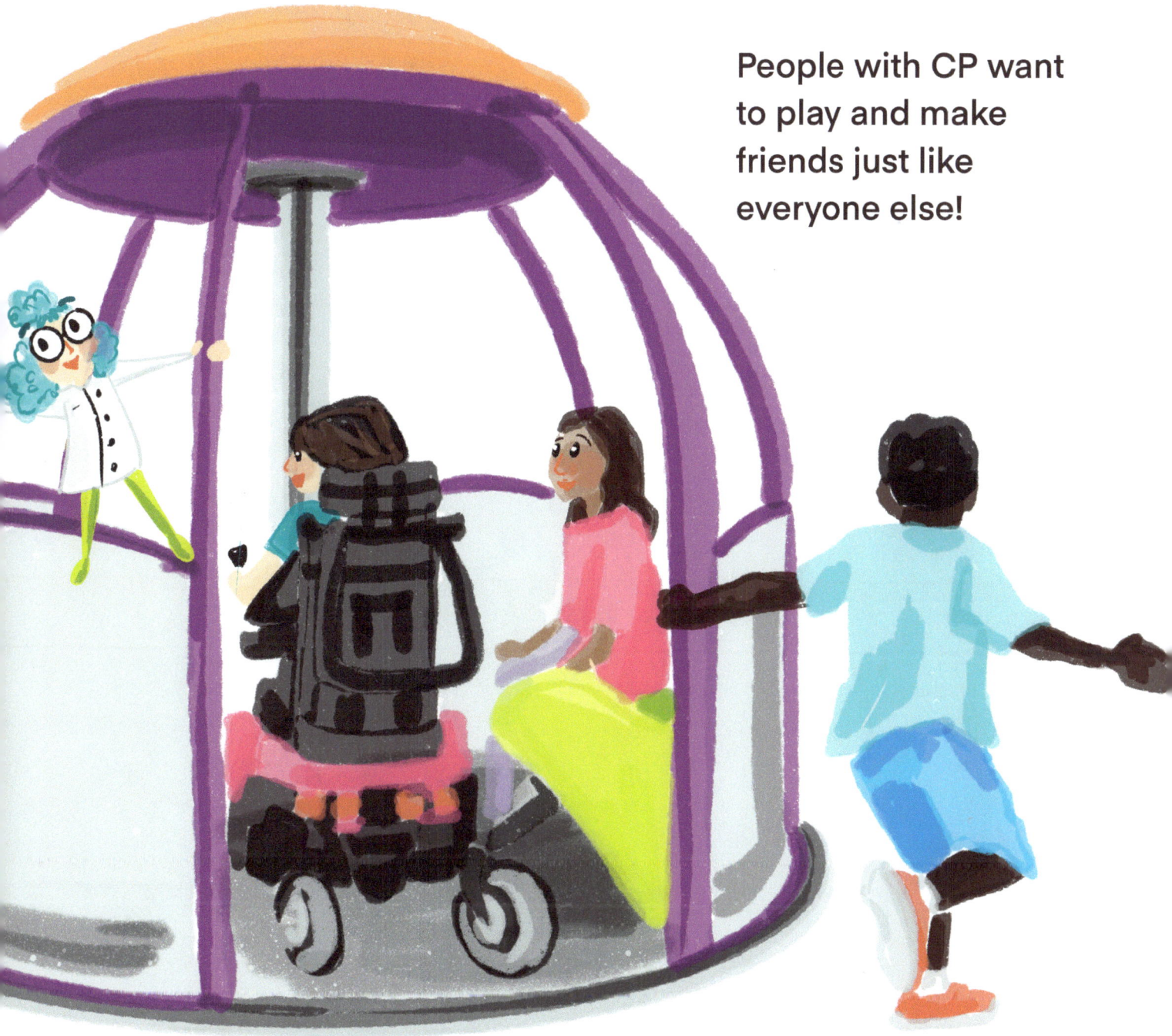

27

Now that you've learned all about Cerebral Palsy, you can help by teaching others about it too!

Thank you for being a great advocate for inclusion!

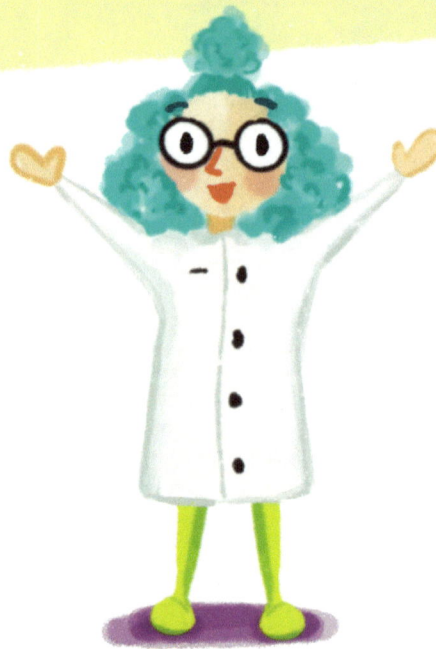

Frequently Asked Questions

What is Cerebral Palsy (CP)?
CP is a medical condition that makes it difficult for a person to control their muscles due to a change in their brain.

How does someone know if they have Cerebral Palsy?
If a parent, caregiver, pediatrician, or other adult, suspects a child may have Cerebral Palsy, the child would likely visit a neurologist. A neurologist is a doctor who studies the nerves and brain and will look at how the child moves. They may also want to take pictures of the child's brain using a big machine called an MRI.

What causes Cerebral Palsy?
CP is caused by abnormal brain development or damage to the developing brain, typically before or during birth, or in early infancy (before age two). This can be a result of genetic mutations that affect brain development, infections during pregnancy, a disruption of blood and/or oxygen to the baby's brain before birth, lack of oxygen during birth, premature birth, brain infections after birth (e.g. meningitis), and/or head injuries. In some cases, the cause of CP is unknown.

How common is Cerebral Palsy?
CP is estimated to occur in about 1 of every 325 children in the United States. Approximately 17 to 18 million people have CP worldwide. Of all children born with CP, 60% are born at term.

Is Cerebral Palsy contagious?
Nope! CP is not contagious like the cold or flu.

Does Cerebral Palsy look the same in everyone?
No. While there are categories to describe CP, every person is impacted slightly

differently. For some people, CP may greatly impact how they move, talk, eat, and/or breathe. For other people, CP is very subtle.

What are the different types of Cerebral Palsy?
There are a few main types of CP:
- Spastic: muscles are stiff and tight
- Dyskinetic: involuntary movements in parts of the body
- Ataxic: poor coordination and balance
- Hypotonic: muscles get tired easily
- Mixed: a combination of two or more types

The most common type of CP is spastic CP. This impacts 80% of all people with CP.

In addition to these four main types, CP can also be classified by the location of the affected body parts.
- Quadriplegia: both arms and both legs
- Hemiplegia: one arm and one leg on the same side of the body
- Diplegia: only both legs or only both arms
- Monoplegia: only one arm or only one leg

So, a person with spastic hemiplegia would have stiff and tight muscles in their arm and leg on one side of their body. A person with ataxic quadriplegia would have poor coordination and balance in both arms and both legs.

Can you cure Cerebral Palsy?
There is no cure for CP, and that's okay! There are things a person with CP can do to make life more comfortable including going to a physical and/or occupational therapist and taking medications that help relax stiff muscles.

How should I talk to someone with Cerebral Palsy? What if they can't talk to me?
People with CP want to be treated with kindness and make friends just like everyone else. Even if someone with CP has difficulty talking, it doesn't mean you should ignore them. Remember, CP describes muscles, not what someone understands. This is why you should always presume competence. Presuming competence means treating people with disabilities as whole people capable of their unique thoughts, opinions, and feelings. It also means that just because someone may show understanding in a different way than you do, does not mean they don't understand.

While someone with CP may not use their voice to talk, they can still communicate. This communication may happen through a computer, buttons they push, sign language, facial expressions, pointing, and so much more!

When is Cerebral Palsy Awareness Month?
March is CP Awareness Month! Wear green (the color of CP awareness) and show your support for those living with CP.

Where can I learn more about Cerebral Palsy?
If you'd like to learn more about CP, consider visiting the websites listed below:

Online Resources:
- Cerebral Palsy Alliance Research Foundation
- Cerebral Palsy Foundation
- United Cerebral Palsy

However, the best way to learn about CP is by talking to someone with CP and asking about their experience. While asking questions is a great way to learn and be more understanding, remember that some people with CP may not be comfortable sharing about their personal lives. That's okay! We are all allowed to choose what we want to talk about. Having a disability does not mean always having to teach others about it.

References

Centers for Disease Control and Prevention. (n.d.). About cerebral palsy. https://www.cdc.gov/cerebral-palsy/about/index.html

Centers for Disease Control and Prevention. (2022, May 2). Data and statistics for Cerebral Palsy. Centers for Disease Control and Prevention. https://archive.cdc.gov/www_cdc_gov/ncbddd/cp/data.html

Cerebral Palsy Alliance Research Foundation (2023). Cerebral palsy facts. https://cparf.org/what-is-cerebral-palsy/facts-about-cerebral-palsy/

Cerebral Palsy Foundation. (n.d.). https://www.yourcpf.org/

Cerebral Palsy Resource. (2025, February 3). https://cpresource.org/